Beat Your Food Yearning: The Secret to Curing Obesity

By

Charles C. Curry

nor full can the document be copied, scanned, faxed, or retained without approval from the publisher or creator.

Table of contents

Chapter 1 2
Speedy Begin to obtain results quickly 2
Bit by bit directions to normally get in shape quickly: 2
Procedures for careful eating include: 2
Chapter 2 2
Improving and accelerating the interaction: 2
Develop Strong Inspirations, Three Insider Facts: 2
The 6 Best Weight Reduction Inspiration Tips: 2
5 Methods for propelling Yourself to Get in shape: 2
Chapter 3 2
Have a recuperation intent to weight reduction 2
Coming up next are the mishap recuperation tips: 2
Following these tips will assist you with recovering ground: 2
Eat what you love yet get thinner: 2
Chapter 4 2
Douse your desires 2
Tips to beat food desires: 2
Look at these tips on the best way to get more fiber in your eating regimen: 2
Characterizing and Estimating Food desire: 2
Conclusion 2
Introduction 1

Introduction

Obesity is the over-the-top or strange amassing of fat or fat tissue in the body that might hinder well-being. Heftiness has turned into a pandemic which has deteriorated throughout the previous 50 years.

Obesity is most apparently driving sort 2 diabetes,

which can have awful results, including visual impairment and foot removals. Be that as it may, it is almost certain to cause other harm as well.

It ought not to be neglected - in spite of the fact that it has been - that corpulence sets individuals at a higher gamble of winding up in serious consideration with Coronavirus.

Expanded Dietary Protein as a Dietary Technique to Forestall or Potentially Treat Stoutness

Heftiness in America keeps on being a significant general well-being concern. Arising logical proof recommends that an eating routine that is a helpful dietary system can forestall good a healthy living as well as treat weight. This paper gives a concise summary of the most recent exploration in regards to the impacts of higher protein diets to further develop body weight the executives and energy consumption guidelines. An explicit spotlight on the impacts of expanded dietary protein on hunger control, satiety, and food desires is additionally investigated.

High protein consumes fewer calories and has acquired both help and analysis over the course of the last ten years when prescribed as a dietary procedure to forestall as well as treat stoutness. Although various examinations have shown enhancements in energy admission guidelines and body weight the board, others hypothesize decreased diet quality and destructive impacts on bone and kidney capability. This paper gives clinical proof supporting the job of higher protein feasts and additionally counts calories in advancing general well-being.

Food Desires

Physiological signs assume a basic part in managing energy consumption during intense as well as constant energy irregularity states. Be that as it may, most Americans are headed to eat through libertine, reward-driven signals set off by the current obesogenic climate, which comprises free and simple admittance to profoundly agreeable, energy-thick food varieties. Information from our lab has as of late demonstrated the way that higher protein feasts can essentially influence reward-driven eating conduct. In these examinations, overweight and stout people consumed either higher or standard protein feasts. Utilizing utilitarian attractive reverberation imaging, we distinguished the brain enactment designs because of food improvements before resulting eating events. Contrasted with standard protein dinners, the higher protein variants prompted diminished actuation in select cortico-limbic cerebrum locales, including the insula or potentially center pre-cerebrum. These locales are ordinarily connected with food desires, food rewards, recollections, considerations, and leader capability. We additionally found that higher protein dinners diminished unfortunate night eating on high-fat or potentially high-sugar food varieties contrasted with standard protein feasts. Albeit the information is restricted, there is some sign that expanded dietary protein decidedly influences reward-driven eating conduct.

High protein eats less carbs have acquired both help and analysis over the course of the last ten years when prescribed as a dietary system to forestall or potentially treat weight. Although various examinations have shown enhancements in energy consumption guidelines and body weight the board, others hypothesize diminished diet quality and destructive consequences for bone and kidney capability. This paper gives clinical proof supporting the job of higher protein dinners and additionally eating less in advancing generally speaking wellbeing. The impacts of expanded dietary protein on hunger control, satiety, and food desires are likewise investigated.

Chapter 1
Speedy Begin to obtain results quickly

Expert and homegrown obligations pass on next to no time for you to investigate your well-being and everyday schedules. Over the long run, this prompts unfortunate propensities like troublesome dinners and having some unacceptable kind of food at some unacceptable time. An immediate consequence of such a way of life is gaining weight.

The way to a solid body according to how much food is a blend of a decent eating routine, exercise and rest, and adjusting to our normal body beat. Our body weight reduction bundle incorporates viable well-being and treatment treatments that utilize spices, treatments, and diet and way of life upgrades with an emphasis on empowering positive propensities for feasible long-haul benefits.

The Program is led in 3 stages

Clean-up:

Begins with detoxification as well as purifying the framework to invigorate digestion.

Nurturing:

Cautiously giving the body the right eating routine and exercise routine took special care of individual necessities.

Maintaining:

Distinguishing and focusing on a solid way of life by outlining a maintainable eating routine and exercise plans alongside homegrown treatments pointed toward further developing metabolic action that clears channels and invigorates the circulatory framework to work on the end of poisons.

Bit by bit directions to normally get in shape quickly:

In this article, we think about 10 powerful techniques for weight reduction:
The Mysterious Ways of Getting More Fit.

The method for weight reduction that logical investigation upholds incorporates the following:

1. Attempting irregular fasting

Irregular fasting is an example of eating that includes customary transient diets and consuming feasts within a more limited time span during the day.

A few examinations have shown that momentary irregular fasting, which is as long as 24 weeks in span, prompts weight reduction in overweight people.

The most well-known crooked fasting methods incorporate the following:

Substitute day fasting: Quick every other day and eat a regular eating routine on non-fasting days. It includes eating only 25-30% of the body's energy needs on fasting days.

The 5:2 Eating regimen: Quick on 2 out of at regular intervals. On fasting days eat 500-600 calories. It is ideal to take on a smart dieting design on non-fasting days and to abstain from indulging.

2. Following your eating routine and exercise

To get thinner, they ought to know about what they eat and drink every day. One investigation discovered that reliable following of actual work assisted with weight reduction. In the interim, a survey concentrated on tracking down a positive connection between weight reduction and the recurrence of checking food admission and exercise. Indeed, even a gadget is really a valuable weight-reduction instrument.

3. Eating carefully

Careful eating is a training where individuals focus on how and where they eat food. These skills can help individuals to benefit from the food they eat and keep a good weight.

As the vast majority have occupied existences, they will quite often eat rapidly on the run, in the vehicle, working in their work areas, and staring at the television. As such, many people are careful of the food they are eating.

Procedures for careful eating include:

1. Plunking down to eat, ideally at a table: Focus on the food and partake in the experience.

2. Keeping away from interruptions while eating: Try not to turn on the television, or a PC or telephone.

3. Eating gradually: Get some margin to bite and enjoy the food.

4. Settling on thoughts about food decisions:

 Pick food varieties that are loaded with sustaining supplements and those that will be fulfilled for quite a long time as opposed to minutes.

5. Having protein for breakfast

Protein can direct hunger chemicals to assist people to feel full.

Scientists noticed that youthful grown-ups have likewise exhibited that the hormonal impacts of having a high-protein breakfast can keep going for a few hours.

6. Scaling back sugar and refined carbs

The Western eating routine is progressively high in

added sugars, which has distinct prompts corpulence, in any event, when the sugar happens in refreshments as opposed to food.

Refined starches are intensely handled food sources that never again contain fiber and different supplements. These include rice, bread, and pasta.

These food variations rush to the procedure, and they convert to glucose quickly.

Where potential, individuals ought to trade handled and sweet food sources for additional invigorating choices. Great food trades include:

spice teas and natural products mixed water rather than high sugar soft drinks smoothies with water or milk rather than natural product juice

7. Eating a lot of fiber

Dietary fiber points out plant-based carbs which are hard to process in the small digestive tract, in contrast to sugar and starch. Remembering a lot of fiber for the eating regimen can expand the emotion of completion, possibly prompting a reduction in weight.

Fiber-rich food sources include:

entire grain breakfast cereals, entire wheat pasta, entire grain bread, oats, grain.

leafy foods

peas, beans, and heartbeats

nuts, and seeds.

8.Adjusting stomach microorganisms

One arising area of examination is zeroing in on the job of microorganisms in the stomach on the weight of the executives.

Each individual has different assortments and measures of organisms that can not be seen with the eyes in their stomach. A few sorts can build how much energy the individual harvests from food, prompting fat testimony and weight gain.

The types of food sources that can expand the quantity of good microscopic organisms in the stomach include:

Matured food sources: These upgrade the capability of good microscopic organisms while restraining the development of awful bacteria. and it additionally contains great measures of probiotics, which help to increment great microbes. Specialists have concentrated broadly, and concentrate on results recommended that it has against weight impacts. Likewise, studies have shown that overcoming your desires might assist with advancing weight reduction in overweight ladies.

Prebiotic food varieties: These invigorate the development and movement of a portion of the great microscopic organisms that help weight control. Prebiotic fiber happens in many products of the soil, particularly onion, garlic, asparagus, leeks, banana, and avocado. It is likewise in grains, like oats and grain.

9. Getting a decent night's rest

Various investigations have shown that getting less than 5-6 hours of rest each night is related to an expanded rate of stoutness. There are a few purposes for this.

The research proposes that deficient or low-quality rest dials back the cycle in which the body changes calories over completely to energy, called digestion. At the point when digestion is less successful, the body might store unused energy as fat. What's more, unfortunately, rest can build the development of insulin and cortisolTrusted Source, which additionally brief fat stockpiling.

10. Dealing with your feelings of anxiety

Stress sets off the arrival of chemicals, for example, adrenaline and cortisol, which at first decline hunger as a feature of the body's survival reaction.

In any case, when individuals are under steady pressure, cortisol can stay in the circulation system for longer, which will expand their hunger and possibly lead to them eating more.

Cortisol flags the need to renew the body's wholesome stores from the favored source carb.

Insulin then, at that point, moves the sugar from starches from the blood to the muscles and cerebrum. On the note that the person doesn't involve this sugar, the body will store it as fat.

Specialists found that carrying out an 8-week stress-the-board mediation program brought about a huge decrease in the weight file of youngsters and teenagers who are overweight or have stoutness.

A few strategies for overseeing pressure include:

contemplation
breathing and unwinding methods
investing some energy outside, for instance, strolling or cultivating.

Why get thinner?

There are so many clarifications behind getting in shape:

Appearance: Certain individuals might feel that assuming they get in shape, they will look more appealing, fitter, or better.

Certainty and self-perception: Certain individuals with abundance weight or corpulence might have an awkward outlook on their appearance.

Generally well-being: Keeping a proper weight can assist with supporting general well-being and forestall sicknesses like sort 2 diabetes.

Explicit circumstances: Side effects of type 2 diabetes, for instance, may improve or disappear when an individual loses overabundance weight.

Fitness: A health improvement plan that includes exercise can leave an individual inclination fitter, with more energy and endurance.

Sports rivalries: In certain games, for example, boxing, an individual might try to control their weight to remain in their current weight classification.

Fertility: Ripeness treatment seems, by all accounts, to be more powerful in ladies with heftiness and polycystic ovary disorder assuming that they lose some weight before treatment.

Chapter 2
Improving and accelerating the interaction:

Develop Strong Inspirations, Three Insider Facts:

1: Compose an Exercise Agreement for Yourself (and Sign It):

Genuinely commit to yourself by mapping out an exercise contract for the week or month - record how frequently each week you will exercise, at what power, and incorporate a few explicit wellness objectives as long as necessary.

Make various awards for accomplishing every one of your agreement objectives. For instance, on the off chance that you meet your recurrence objective (the number of days you focus on working out each week), you procure a $25 gift voucher for your #1 store. On the off chance that you meet your objective of removing an inch from your midsection estimation, you procure another set of exercise pants. On the off chance that you meet your MEP objective, partake in a back rub.

In the wake of drafting the agreement complete with explicit prizes, sign it like you would a legitimately restricting record. Consider yourself responsible for the agreement, and unquestionably offer yourself the prizes en route!

2: Make a Wellness Vision:

You can make your wellness vision in more than one way. On the off chance that you're an essayist, you can compose your wellness vision in story structure. Assuming you're a craftsman, you can draw or shape your wellness vision. On the off chance that you're a performer, you can sing about your wellness vision. Making a wellness vision incorporates portraying how you will feel, look, and go about because of accomplishing your exercise objectives. Carve out the opportunity to obviously recognize your particular wellness or exercise objectives and truly ponder how you will feel, look, and go about because of accomplishing your objectives. It resembles making the most ideal adaptation representing things to come to you!

Partake all the while and return to your wellness vision frequently for motivation.

3: Begin Jabber with your Social Associations, Empowering discussion

with your social associations.

Look at how your buddies are doing their exercises and proposition them some sure criticism about their advancement.

Make sure to questions or request exhortation. On the off chance that you see a social association that is procuring the sort of errand, you need to procure, connect, and inquire as to whether they have any exhortation.

The 6 Best Weight Reduction Inspiration Tips:

Master tips to assist you with getting inspired and remain as such:

1: Plan an Arrangement that Suits Your Way of life:

Make your own arrangement so it will squeeze into the manner in which you live. In principle, you want to remove simply 150 calories every day to shed 15 pounds in a year, so begin little to have a superior opportunity to keep up with your weight reduction inspiration.

Contemplate the food varieties you can — and can't — live without, then attempt to construct your arrangement around them. On the off chance that you're a conceived snacker, partition your day-to-day calories into six or seven small dinners so you generally feel like you're having a snack. Anything that you do, don't surrender your number one food variety. You'll unavoidably feel denied, which will just make your desires more grounded — and your determination more fragile.

2: Put Your Arrangement In writing:

Any effective endeavor requires an arrangement that portrays its central goal and points of interest on the best way to accomplish it — without one, you have no clue about where you're beginning, where you're going, or the way in which you'll arrive. Begin by posting every one of the reasons you can imagine for thinning down — at the end of the day, characterize your weight reduction inspiration on paper. Whenever you've decided precisely the exact thing you need to accomplish and your cutoff time, work in reverse to make a month-to-month strategy with sensible and explicit objectives for shedding pounds, (for example, focusing on solid eating).

3: Keep Your Commitments:

Assuming you're battling to stay with your weight reduction inspiration, practice honesty in different aspects of your life, and Work on staying with commitments or responsibilities you've made in different parts of your life to reinforce your own subliminal conviction that you can maintain the guarantee to shed pounds that you've made to yourself.

4: Avoid Examinations:

Sticking and posting pictures of supermodels might seem like great weight reduction inspiration, yet as per research, harming your progress is almost certain.

Rather than contrasting yourself with unreasonable style models, remain propelled by posting pictures of you at your best for a serious portion of weight reduction motivation.

5: Center Around an Inclination:

Time and again we get baffled by zeroing in on a particular number on the scale, or even an errand we should do to arrive at our objective, (for example, working out), which is a fast method for destroying your zing.

Focus on your temperament after you've eaten a good dinner or how you feel after an incredible exercise — weight reduction inspiration doesn't necessarily need to precede an action,

In the event that you center around how you feel each time you work out, you'll get every one of the advantages of consuming calories, in addition to the support of recollecting how great it felt to make it happen, which ought to build your inspiration to accomplish more.

6: Drape Your Inspiration By the Mirror:

Showing off an exceptional piece of your closet is an incredible everyday weight reduction motivation. Pick something you'll anticipate wearing and hang it near your mirror. I envision myself wearing it and ponder how great I will feel, Since it's a thing you currently own or want to wear, it's much doubtful to be a ridiculous objective and will assist with spiking your inspiration to continue to go to the exercise center.

Computerize inspiration Right now Of drive:

What inspires you to get more fit can differ from one individual to another. Be that as it may, finding your inspiration can include recognizing the reasons you need to get fitter, setting your assumptions, and tracking down help. Beginning and adhering to a sound weight-reduction plan can some of the time appear to be unthinkable.

Frequently, individuals essentially miss the mark on inspiration to get everything rolling or lose their inspiration to continue onward.

This article examines 5 methods for rousing yourself to get thinner:

5 Methods for propelling Yourself to Get in shape:

What spurs you to get more fit can fluctuate from one individual to another. In any case, finding your inspiration can include recognizing the reasons you need to shed pounds, setting your assumptions, and tracking down help.

Beginning and adhering to a sound weight-reduction plan can now and then appear to be incomprehensible.

1. Make a decision Why You Need to Get in shape:

Obviously, characterize every one of the reasons you need to get more fit and record them on paper. This will help you with maintenance, commitment, and persuasion to arrive at your weight loss objectives.

Attempt to peruse them day to day and use them as an update when enticed to wander from your weight reduction plans.

Your reasons could incorporate forestalling diabetes, staying aware of grandkids, putting your best self forward for an occasion, working on your fearlessness, or squeezing into a specific set of pants.

Many individuals begin getting in shape on the

grounds that their primary care physician recommended it, however, research shows that individuals are more effective assuming their weight reduction inspiration comes from the inside.

2. Have Sensible Assumptions:

Many eating regimens and diet items grant speedy and easy weight loss. Be that as it may, most specialists suggest just shedding 1-2 pounds (0.5-1 kg) each week.

Putting forth impossible objectives can prompt sensations of disappointment and influence you to surrender. In actuality, putting forth and achieving feasible objectives prompts sensations of achievement.

A review utilizing information from a few weight reduction focuses found that ladies who expected to lose the most weight were probably going to exit the program. Fortunately, only a tad weight reduction of 5-10% of your body weight can to a great extent affect your well-being. Assuming you are 180 pounds (82 kg), that is only 9-18 pounds (4-8 kg).

Losing 5-10% of your body weight can, as a matter of fact:

Further, develop glucose control

Decrease the gamble of coronary illness

Lower cholesterol levels

Decrease joint agony

Decrease the gamble of specific diseases

3.   Center   around Interaction Objectives:

Many individuals attempting to get more fit just put forth result objectives, or objectives they need to achieve toward the end.

Ordinarily, a result objective will be your last objective weight.

All things being equal, you ought to put forth process objectives, or what moves you will make to arrive at your ideal result. An illustration of an interaction objective is practicing four times each week.

Laying out shrewd interaction objectives will assist you with remaining persuaded, while zeroing in just on result objectives can prompt disillusionment and lessen your inspiration.

4. Pick an Arrangement That Accommodates Your Way of life:

Find a weight reduction plan that you can adhere to, and stay away from plans that would be almost difficult to continue in the long haul.

While there are many various eating regimens, most depend on cutting calories.

Decreasing your calorie admission will prompt weight reduction, yet slimming down, particularly continuously yo eating less junk food, has been viewed as an indicator of future weight gain.

Along these lines, keep away from severe weight control plans that totally wipe out specific food varieties. Research has observed that those with a win-big or bust outlook are less inclined to shed weight.

Everything being equal, try to consider making your own main arrangement.

The accompanying dietary propensities have been demonstrated to assist you with shedding weight:

Diminishing calorie consumption

Lessening segment sizes:

Lessening the recurrence of bites

Lessening seared food and pastries

Counting foods grown from the ground.

Pick an eating plan that you can adhere to:

The long haul and stay away from an outrageous or convenient solution that counts calories.

5. Try not to Go for the gold Excuse Yourself:

You don't need to be amazing to get more fit.

Assuming you have a win big or bust approach, you're less inclined to accomplish your objectives.

At the point when you are excessively prohibitive, you might end up saying "I had a burger and fries for lunch, so I should have pizza for supper." All things being equal, attempt to say, "I had a major lunch, so I ought to hold back nothing supper".

Furthermore, try not to thrash yourself when you commit an error. Foolish contemplations will simply obstruct your inspiration:

All things considered, pardon yourself. Recollect

that one mix-up won't destroy your advancement. At the point when you hold back nothing, will rapidly lose your inspiration. By permitting yourself adaptability and pardoning yourself, you can remain spurred all through your weight reduction venture.

Chapter 3
Have a recuperation intent to weight reduction

Lessen your everyday calorie consumption by 200 calories, except if this places you in a reach that is excessively low for good well-being. Steadily increment your everyday workout time by 15 to 30 minutes. In the event that is conceivable, likewise, increment the force. Center around three-to-four-week patterns in weight reduction rather than day-to-day changes.

Coming up next are the mishap recuperation tips:

1. Levels:

Hitting plateaus is ordinary. The vast majority arrive at one following a half year of weight reduction.

Attempt these arrangements:

Survey your food and movement records to ensure you haven't allowed yourself to backtrack with bigger segments or less activity.

Diminish your day-to-day calorie consumption by 200 calories, except if this places you in a reach that is excessively low for good well-being.

Progressively increment your everyday workout time by 15 to 30 minutes. In the event that is conceivable, likewise increment the power.

Center around three-to-four-week patterns in weight reduction rather than day-to-day changes.

Reevaluate your program and objectives. Assuming that it's an excessive amount to diminish calories or increment movement, it's smarter to be happy with the weight you have lost than to tap out and recover it.

2. Managing slips:

A pass happens when you return to your old ways of behaving for a brief time. In the event that few slips have happened in a brief time frame, it's enticing to think your weight-reduction plan is excessively difficult. No real reason to stress; a slip-by is only a transient obstacle.

Following these tips will assist you with recovering ground:

Try not to allow bad reflection to dominate. Botches occur, and every day is an opportunity to begin once more.

Make another little stride. Changing your life doesn't occur at the same time. Remember that changing ways of behaving in little ways can amount to a major contrast in your life.

Request and acknowledge support. Tolerating support from others is certainly not an indication of a shortcoming, nor does it imply that you're falling flat. Get support from others when you have troublesome days.

Plan your system. Obviously, distinguish the issue, and afterward make a rundown of potential arrangements. On the off chance that one arrangement doesn't work, attempt one more until you find one that does.

Sort out your disappointment with working out. Keep it energetic and, surprisingly, fun — don't involve actual work as a discipline.

3. Commit once again to your objectives:

Audit them to ensure they're as yet sensible.

In spite of the fact that omissions can be

frustrating, they can likewise show you a great deal. Maybe your objectives are ridiculous or certain systems don't work. In particular, understand that all trust isn't lost when you pass. Simply re-energize your inspiration, commit once again to your program, and return to sound ways of behaving.

Eat what you love yet get thinner:

With regards to accomplishing and keeping a sound weight, you could think you need to quit any pretense of eating what you love. Yet, that isn't true. It's feasible to eat your number one food source yet accomplish your weight reduction objectives.

Here is a speedy aide on eating with some restraint and fulfilling your desires:

1. Segment control:

Maybe the main step of all in having the option to eat what you love comes down to partition control. In the New Mayo Center Eating regimen program, you'll realize about solid part estimates. This could take some becoming accustomed to, however, it tends to be an enlightening encounter to find what a fitting piece size truly is. What's more, when you begin rehearsing segment control and start eating the right food sources in the perfect sums you'll before long observe that a little serving of your number one treat is all you really want.

You'll likewise learn stunts all through the program that will assist with keeping you from indulging. For instance:

1.Attempt to try not to eat food sources directly from the bundle which makes crunching on numerous servings generally excessively simple:

All things being equal, dole up a solitary serving and afterward place the bundle concealed.

2. Appreciate the flavor

At the point when you eat your #1 food sources, rather than gobbling up them in thoughtless swallows, attempt to dial back and permit yourself to partake in the occasion, relishing every single chomp, as a matter of fact. Careful eating is another ability you'll acquire in this book Diet Program.

A great method for rehearsing careful eating is with a piece of chocolate:

1. Plunk down and take each little nibble in turn. Save each chomp in your mouth for a couple of seconds prior to gulping.

2. Notice the rich flavor, smooth surface, and extreme pleasantness. You wouldn't believe how one little piece of chocolate can fulfill a sugar hankering when enjoyed gradually.

3. Add development and exercise to your day. Practice accompanies numerous medical advantages that range from easing pressure and further developing memory to assisting you with resting better. Yet, with regards to weight the board, the genuine reward is the acceleration of your calorie consumption. Realizing that you're consuming a couple of additional calories permits you to partake in a most loved food sometimes while you're wanting it. Anything that active work you pick, do it reliably. As well as assisting with weight reduction, exercise can assist with further developing satisfaction and furthermore make the right attitude for eating better. There are a lot of extraordinary activities you can do right from your home.

4. Top off on foods grown from the ground first.

Products of the soil can be extraordinary supplements to the food sources you love. In addition to the fact that they are low in calories, they keep you feeling full and fulfilled. Thus, with regards to adjusting your sustenance, consistently attempt to top off on nutritious food varieties by beginning with vegetables and organic products. As opposed to eating your number one treat while starving, eat a good feast first and save the candy for dessert. You're probably going to eat less sweets. Furthermore, by saving the sugar for after your dinner, you'll assist with forestalling your glucose levels from spiking. Adding products of the soil to your eating routine is an enduring, significant propensity that will assist you with living the best rendition of your life. The New Mayo Facility Diet includes a new, intuitive Propensity Enhancer that makes building better propensities very much like this one fun!

5. Cook the better variant of what you love.

Once in a while, your #1 solace food varieties simply need a little change to a great extent to become better — however similarly as scrumptious — renditions of themselves. For example, you could consider changing how you cook specific fixings: Rather than profoundly broiling food varieties, attempt air-searing them! One more extraordinary.

method for overhauling what you're longing for is by trading for better fixings:

Have a go at going to natural products as a wellspring of pleasantness in baking as opposed to sugar. All you really want is a receptive outlook and a readiness to try in the kitchen.

Chapter 4
Douse your desires

The word reference meaning of desire is this:
I. To really want.
ii. To desperately require; require.
iii. To ask genuinely for; implore.
Can we just look at things objectively, we as a whole get food desires, and when they strike it tends to be

almost difficult to simply say no. By giving in you're possibly adding huge calories that can include no doubt. Subsequent to fulfilling a hankering, sensations of culpability and overcome frequently follow.

For what reason are desires so enticing around evening time?

Generally, we partner evening time with endlessly unwinding with eating. It is our chance to slow down and prize ourselves following a long and depleting day. Since we are in a casual state and maybe not as zeroed in on solid ways of behaving as we are over the course of the day, it is bound to enjoy solace food varieties, for example, treats, frozen yogurt, and chips. Now is the ideal time to stop the evening frenzy — here's a manual to assist with beating those desires and remaining fixed on your weight reduction objectives!

Tips to beat food desires:

1.   Eat little and continuous feasts to forestall spikes in hunger: Following a steady eating design with accentuation on protein will keep you feeling full, making it more straightforward to beat those late-night desires.

2. Consume a lot of fiber: Fiber-containing food varieties make mass and leave you feeling satisfied for a significant stretch of time. Pick high-fiber snacks with protein to get the most value for your calorie money.

Look at these tips on the best way to get more fiber in your eating regimen:

I. Try not to keep activating the origin of food in the house:
Out of the picture and therefore irrelevant! Give your kitchen a makeover and just keep sound snacks around. On the occasion a food hankering goes along, there might be sound choices to browse.

2. Keep yourself occupied:
An adjustment of routine can assist with warding off desires. Change everything around! Ditch the television remote and have a go at something new and

significant. Join a book club, pursue yoga classes, get up to speed with messages, begin a blog, or do a home exercise video to keep involved and zero in on things other than food.

3. If conceivable, utilize the DVR on your TV:

Pre-record your #1 shows with the goal that you can quickly forward through plugs and stay away from on-screen food allurements.

4. Make non-food compensations for practicing good eating habits:

As opposed to indulging yourself with a bowl of your #1 frozen yogurt, enjoy a mani-pedi, knead, or new exercise top on days where you tried sincerely and merit a little treat. Other more affordable choices incorporate a free wellness class, stroll around the area, or air pocket shower.

5. If all else fails, yield to a solid tidbit:

While numerous food desires result from natural upgrades, some may be obtained from genuine cravings. One portion of carrying on with a solid way of life is having the option to pay attention to your body. Assuming your body is letting you know that it's eager and requires fuel, don't overlook it.

6. Make a point to pick a high protein nibble to forestall extra desires and consistently drink a lot of water to keep from indulging late evening:

Characterizing and Estimating Food desire:

Food desire is much of the time characterized as a powerful urge to eat. Much work has shown that it reliably and tentatively predicts eating and weight-related results, adding to the developing heftiness pandemic. In spite of the fact that there are clear distinctions in sexual orientation in the pervasiveness and well-being outcomes of stoutness, somewhat minimal ongoing work has examined distinctions in sexual orientation in desiring, or any sex-chemical-based contrasts as they connect with periods of the monthly cycle. Here, we recommend that orientation-related contrasts in food hankering add to orientation-related contrasts in stoutness. Attracting on discoveries the compulsion writing, we feature ways of integrating orientation-based contrasts in food hankering into treatment draws near, possibly working on the viability of heftiness and weight reduction treatment. In general, this survey means to underscore the significance of exploring distinctions in sexual orientation in food hankering, with a view towards educating the improvement regarding more compelling medicines for heftiness and weight reduction.

Mainstream society frequently depicts distinctions in sexual orientation in food desires, for example, the idea that men pine for exquisite food varieties (e.g., burgers) while ladies long for sweet food sources (e.g., chocolate), particularly as they approach menses. While this isn't generally the situation, some examination has upheld distinctions in sexual orientation in the sort of food longed for, yet additionally in clinically significant qualities of desire like recurrence, seriousness, and guidelines of food desire. In the areas underneath, we will initially characterize desires and examine how food desire can anticipate eating and weight gain. We will then, at that point, contend that because of this prescient relationship, desire is a possible illustrative component for quickly expanding paces of corpulence, which is the subsequent driving reason for preventable sickness and demise in the US. Then, we will survey key discoveries on distinctions in sexual orientation in food hankering, and make sense of how these distinctions might underlie distinctions in sexual orientation in stoutness and heftiness-related well-being outcomes. Then, at that point, we will talk about proof that hormonal contrasts among people, and hormonal varieties across ladies' feminine cycles add to such contrasts. At last, attracting discoveries the illicit drug habits writing, we will feature significant ramifications of distinctions in sexual orientation in food hankering for heftiness exploration and treatment. experienced by in excess of 90% of the populace. A few kinds of food hankering are regularly characterized and contemplated. Tonic desire mirrors a general inclination that is capable either over the long haul or in a specific second, without any ecological improvements. It is in many cases connected with forbearance from a specific food and is regularly estimated with multi-thing self-report scales/surveys, including the Food desire Stock. By the way, tonic desire isn't equivalent to hunger, and can be knowledgeable about the shortfall of caloric need. Reasonable cross-over of ordinarily characterized types of food hankering. Schematic and calculated portrayal of the cross-over in definitions and kinds of hankering. Sign-incited hankering is an intense time of hankering, evoked by natural/outside improvements. State hankering is a sensation of hankering in a specific second, whether or not a prompt is available. Characteristic desire alludes to a propensity to feel desire overall; it can allude to hankering every day both within the sight of signals and without prompts. Sizes of the air pockets reflect definitional cross-over across Time and Signal aspects.

Then again, prompt-incited desire is an intense time of hankering, evoked by ecological/outer boosts. In light of such upgrades, people report their ongoing degree of desire , either on a multi-thing scale or a solitary-thing reaction. A huge collection of studies has reliably shown that openness to visual, olfactory, or taste prompts of remarkable food things brings about sign-initiated desire, alongside expansions in fringe physiological signals, for example, pulse, gastric movement, and salivation, known as prompt reactivity. For example, remember to assume a focal part in inspiration and learning, Albeit these mind districts have novel and shifted capabilities, together they structure part of a circuit that distinguishes and encodes the notability of remuneration. Further, the initiation of these locales corresponds with a self-revealed sign-incited hankering. In that capacity, sign-prompted hankering is a molded reaction, wherein food signals present at the hour of food utilization became related to the compensation of eating, and over the long run come to evoke molded physiological, brain, and hankering reactions.

Conclusion

The utilization of higher protein eats less carbs, containing between 25-30% of calorie admission as protein, prompts critical upgrades in body weight the board, through deliberate decreases in energy consumption, weight reduction, and useful changes in body structure. One system of activity is expected, to some extent, to upgrade craving control, satiety, and prize-driven eating conduct. Until now, the base measure of protein expected to get these robotic reactions is 30g of protein/eating event, which is roughly 1½ servings of great protein-rich food varieties. Further, no information exists recommending that this amount of protein utilization evokes any hurtful consequences for kidney and bone well-being. In outline, this

information delineates that
an eating routine wealthy
in protein gives off an
impression of being an
ideal technique to forestall
or potentially treat obesity.